Objective setting is wherever in our reality. We set objectives for our vocations, our wellbeing, and our lives by and large. It appears to be current society is continually reassuring us to consider the following achievement. Nonetheless, what we don't think about enough is the science and technique of how to achieve your objectives. That is the thing that this guide is here to do.

Regardless of whether you're defining individual objectives or expert objectives, this guide will disclose all that you have to know. You can tap the connections underneath to hop to a specific segment or essentially look down to understand everything. Toward the finish of this page, you'll locate a total rundown of the apparent multitude of articles I have composed on objective setting.

I. What is Goal Setting?

Specialists characterize objective setting as the demonstration of choosing an objective or target you wish to accomplish. Sufficiently reasonable. That definition bodes well, however I think there is a substantially more valuable approach to consider defining objectives.

What is Goal Setting?

Most objective setting practices start with an overpaid advisor remaining by a whiteboard and asking something like, "What does achievement resemble to you? In quite certain terms, what would you like to accomplish?"

On the off chance that we are not kidding about accomplishing our objectives, in any case, we should begin with a vastly different inquiry. Instead of thinking about what sort of progress we need, we ought to solicit, "What sort of torment do I need?"

This is a methodology I gained from my companion and creator, Mark Manson. What Mark has acknowledged is that having an objective is the simple part. Who wouldn't have any desire to compose a top of the line book or get thinner or win more cash? Everyone needs to accomplish these objectives.

The genuine test isn't deciding whether you need the outcome, however in the event that you are eager to acknowledge the penances needed to accomplish your objective. Do you need the way of life that accompanies your mission? Do you need the exhausting and appalling cycle that precedes the energizing and marvelous result?

It's anything but difficult to lounge around and figure what we could do or what we'd prefer to do. It is an altogether extraordinary thing to acknowledge the tradeoffs that accompany our objectives. Everyone needs a gold award. Not many individuals need to prepare like an Olympian.

This carries us to our first key understanding. Objective setting isn't just about picking the prizes you need to appreciate, yet in addition the costs you are happy to pay.

Rudders and Oars

Envision a little dinghy. Your objectives resemble the rudder on the pontoon. They set the heading and figure out where you go. In the event that you focus on one objective, at that point the rudder waits and you keep pushing ahead. On the off chance that you flip-flop between objectives, at that point the rudder moves all around and it is anything but difficult to end up paddling around and around.

Nonetheless, there is another piece of the pontoon that is significantly more significant than the rudder: The paddles. In the event that the rudder is your objective, at that point the paddles are your cycle for accomplishing it. While the rudder decides your heading, the paddles decide your advancement.

This similitude of the rudder and the paddles explains the contrast among frameworks and objectives. It is a significant differentiation that shows up wherever throughout everyday life.

In case you're a mentor, you will probably win a title. Your framework is the thing that your group does at training every day.

In case you're an essayist, you will probably compose a book. Your framework is the composing plan that you follow every week.

In case you're a sprinter, you will likely run a long distance race. Your framework is your preparation plan for the month.

In case you're a business person, you will probably manufacture a million dollar business. Your framework is your deals and showcasing measure.

Objectives are helpful for setting the heading. Frameworks are incredible for really gaining ground. Indeed, the essential advantage of having an objective is that it mentions to you what kind of framework you have to set up. Notwithstanding, the framework itself is the thing that really accomplished the outcomes.

This carries us to our second key knowledge. Objectives decide your course. Frameworks decide your advancement. You'll never go anyplace just by holding the rudder. You need to push.

II. Step by step instructions to Set Goals You'll Actually Follow

Okay, since we've examined the tradeoffs and frameworks that accompany objectives, we should discuss how to set objectives you'll really follow.

There are three fundamental systems I like to utilize when objective setting. We should discuss every one at this point.

1. Savagely Eliminate Your Goals

Therapists have an idea they allude to as "objective rivalry."

Objective rivalry says that probably the best hindrance to accomplishing your objectives is different objectives you have. At the end of the day, your objectives are rivaling each other for your time and consideration. At whatever point you pursue another objective, you need to pull center and vitality from your different interests. This is essentially The Four Burners Theory in real life. At the point when you turn one burner up, you need to turn others down.

Presently, there is uplifting news. Perhaps the quickest approaches to gain ground on your objectives is to just press delay on less significant things and spotlight on each objective in turn. Here and there you simply need to redesign your needs a smidgen and out of nowhere progress comes substantially more rapidly in light of the fact that you are presently completely dedicated to an objective that was just getting moderate consideration beforehand.

This is a significant knowledge. Normally, when we neglect to arrive at our objectives, we think something wasn't right with our objective or our methodology. Specialists let us know, "You have to think greater! Pick a fantasy that is so huge it will inspire you consistently." Or we let ourselves know, "If just I had more hours in the day!"

These reasons cloud the greater issue. What regularly resembles an issue of objective setting is really an issue of objective determination. What we truly need isn't greater objectives, yet better core interest. You have to pick a certain something and heartlessly dispose of everything else. In the expressions of Seth Godin, "You needn't bother with additional time, you simply need to choose."

Our lives resemble flower hedges. As a flower shrubbery develops, it makes a bigger number of buds than it can continue. On the off chance that you converse with an accomplished nursery worker, they will disclose to you that flower hedges should be pruned to draw out the best in both their appearance and their exhibition. As such, on the off chance that you need a flower hedge to flourish, at that point you have to remove a portion of the great buds so the extraordinary ones can completely bloom.

Our objectives are comparable. They should be reliably pruned and cut down. It's normal for new objectives to come into our lives and to get amped up for new chances—simply like it's normal for a flower hedge to include new buds. In the event that we can marshal the fortitude to prune away a couple of our objectives, at that point we make the space we requirement for the rest of the objectives to completely bloom. Full development and ideal living require pruning.

I've expounded on an assortment of procedures for getting your needs all together and concentrating on each thing in turn, including:

The Ivy Lee Method

Warren Buffett's 25-5 Rule

The Eisenhower Box

The 20 Slot Rule

The Myth of Multitasking

Investigate those procedures and evaluate one that impacts you.

2. Stack Your Goals

Examination has indicated that you are 2x to 3x bound to adhere to your objectives on the off chance that you make a particular arrangement for when, where, and how you will play out the conduct. For instance, in one examination researchers requested that individuals round out this sentence: "During the following week, I will participate in any event 20 minutes of overwhelming activity on [DAY] at [TIME OF DAY] at/in [PLACE]."

Scientists found that individuals who rounded out this sentence were 2x to 3x bound to really practice contrasted with a benchmark group who didn't make arrangements for their future conduct. Clinicians call these particular plans "usage goals" since they state when, where, and how you expect to execute a specific conduct. This finding has been rehashed across many investigations and has been found to build the chances that individuals will begin working out, start reusing, stay with considering, and even quit smoking.

One of my preferred approaches to use this finding is with a methodology I call propensity stacking. To utilize propensity stacking, simply round out this sentence:

After/Before [CURRENT HABIT], I will [NEW HABIT].

Here are a few models:

Reflection: After I mix my morning espresso, I will think for one moment.

Pushups: Before I clean up, I will complete 10 pushups.

Flossing: After I put my toothbrush down, I will floss my teeth.

Appreciation: Before I have supper, I will say one thing I am thankful for that day.

Systems administration: After I come back from my mid-day break, I will send one email to somebody I need to meet.

Propensity stacking functions admirably in light of the fact that you not just make a particular arrangement for when and where you will actualize your objectives, yet additionally interface your new objectives to something you are as of now doing every day. You can peruse more on the most proficient method to stack propensities and set triggers for your objectives in my famous guide, Transform Your Habits.

I discover this to be a useful method to overcome any issues among objectives and frameworks. Our objectives mention to us what we need to accomplish while our frameworks are the cycle we follow every day. Propensity stacking and usage aims assist us with moving from the objective in our minds to the particular cycle that will make it a reality.

3. Set an Upper Bound

At whatever point we set objectives, we quite often center around the lower bound. That is, we consider the base limit we need to hit. The understood supposition that is, "Hello, in the event that you can accomplish more than the base, pull out all the stops."

An individual may state, "I need to lose at any rate 5 pounds this month."

A business visionary may state, "I need to make at any rate 10 deals calls today."

A craftsman may state, "I need to compose at any rate 500 words today."

A ball player may state, "I need to make in any event 50 free tosses today."

In any case, what might it resemble in the event that we added an upper bound to our objectives and practices?

"I need to lose at any rate 5 pounds this month, yet not more than 10."

"I need to make in any event 10 deals calls today, yet not more than 20."

Disregard Setting Goals.
Concentrate on This Instead.

Winning astuteness asserts that the most ideal approach to accomplish what we need throughout everyday life—improving shape, constructing a fruitful business, loosening up more and stressing less, investing more energy with loved ones—is to set explicit, noteworthy objectives.

For a long time, this was the manner by which I moved toward my propensities as well. Every one was an objective to be reached. I set objectives for the evaluations I needed to get in school, for the loads I needed to lift in the rec center, for the benefits I needed to acquire in business. I prevailing at a couple, yet I fizzled at a ton of them. Inevitably, I started to understand that my outcomes had almost no to do with the objectives I set and about everything to do with the frameworks I followed.

In case you're a mentor, your objective may be to win a title. Your framework is the manner in which you enlist players, deal with your associate mentors, and lead practice.

In case you're a business person, your objective may be to fabricate a million-dollar business. Your framework is the manner by which you test item thoughts, enlist workers, and run promoting efforts.

In case you're an artist, your objective may be to play another piece. Your framework is the means by which frequently you practice, how you separate and tackle troublesome measures, and your technique for getting criticism from your teacher.

Presently for the intriguing inquiry: on the off chance that you totally overlooked your objectives and concentrated distinctly on your framework, OK despite everything succeed? For instance, in the event that you were a ball mentor and you disregarded your objective to win a title and concentrated distinctly on what your group does at training every day, OK despite everything get results?

I figure you would.

The objective in any game is to get done with the best score, yet it is ludicrous to spend the entire game gazing at the scoreboard. The best way to really win is to show signs of improvement every day. In the expressions of three-time Super Bowl victor Bill Walsh, "The score deals with itself." The equivalent is valid for different everyday issues. In the event that you need better outcomes, at that point disregard defining objectives. Concentrate on your framework.

I don't get my meaning by this? Are objectives totally pointless? Obviously not. Objectives are useful for setting a course, yet frameworks are best for gaining ground. A modest bunch of issues emerge when you invest a lot of energy pondering your objectives and insufficient time structuring your frameworks.

Issue #1: Winners and washouts have similar objectives.

Objective setting experiences a genuine instance of survivorship inclination. We focus on the individuals who wind up winning—the survivors—and erroneously expect that eager objectives prompted their prosperity while ignoring the entirety of the individuals who had a similar goal yet didn't succeed.

Each Olympian needs to win a gold award. Each up-and-comer needs to land the position. What's more, in the event that effective and ineffective individuals share similar objectives, at that point the objective can't be what separates the champs from the washouts. It wasn't the objective of winning the Tour de France that impelled the British Cyclists to the head of the game. Probably, they had needed to win the race each prior year—simply like each other expert group. The objective had consistently been there. It was just when they executed an arrangement of persistent little upgrades that they accomplished an alternate result.

Issue #2: Achieving an objective is just a flitting change.

Envision you have an untidy room and you set an objective to clean it. In the event that you gather the vitality to clean up, at that point you will have a tidy up room—for the present. Yet, in the event that you keep up a similar messy, collector propensities that prompted an untidy room in any case, soon you'll be taking a gander at another heap of messiness and seeking after another explosion of inspiration. You're left pursuing a similar result since you never changed the framework behind it. You treated a manifestation without tending to the reason.

Accomplishing an objective just transforms yourself for the occasion. That is the nonsensical thing about progress. We think we have to change our outcomes, yet the outcomes are not the issue. What we truly need to change are the frameworks that cause those outcomes. At the point when you tackle issues at the outcomes level, you just unravel them incidentally. So as to improve for good, you have to take care of issues at the frameworks level. Fix the sources of info and the yields will fix themselves.

Issue #3: Goals confine your bliss.

The verifiable supposition behind any objective is this: "When I arrive at my objective, at that point I'll be glad." The issue with an objectives first attitude is that you're constantly postponing satisfaction until the following achievement. I've slipped into this snare so often I've lost tally. For a considerable length of time, satisfaction was continually something for my future self to appreciate. I guaranteed myself that once I increased twenty pounds of muscle or after my business was included in the New York Times, at that point I could at last unwind.

Moreover, objectives make an "either-or" strife: possibly you accomplish your objective and are fruitful or you fall flat and you are a failure. You intellectually confine yourself to a limited rendition of satisfaction. This is confused. It is impossible that your genuine way through life will coordinate the specific excursion you had as a top priority when you set out. It looks bad to limit your fulfillment to one situation when there are numerous ways to progress.

A frameworks first attitude gives the remedy. At the point when you become hopelessly enamored with the cycle as opposed to the item, you don't need to hold on to allow yourself to be upbeat. You can be fulfilled whenever your framework is running. What's more, a framework can be effective in a wide range of structures, not simply the one you first imagine.

Issue #4: Goals are at chances with long haul progress.

At last, an objective situated mentality can make a "yo-yo" impact. Numerous sprinters buckle down for a considerable length of time, yet when they cross the end goal, they quit preparing. The race is no longer there to propel them. When the entirety of your difficult work is centered around a specific objective, what is left to push you forward after you accomplish it? This is the reason numerous individuals wind up returning to their old propensities in the wake of achieving an objective.

The reason for defining objectives is to dominate the match. The reason for building frameworks is to keep playing the game. Genuine long haul believing is objective less reasoning. It's not about any single achievement. It is about the pattern of unending refinement and consistent improvement. Eventually, it is your pledge to the cycle that will decide your advancement.

The Downside of Work-Life Balance

One approach to consider work-life offset is with an idea known as The Four Burners Theory. Here's the manner by which it was first disclosed to me:

Envision that your life is spoken to by an oven with four burners on it. Every burner represents one significant quadrant of your life.

The main burner speaks to your family.

The subsequent burner is your companions.

The third burner is your wellbeing.

The fourth burner is your work.

The Four Burners Theory says that "so as to be effective you need to cut off one of your burners. Also, so as to be extremely effective you need to cut off two."

Three Views of the Four Burners

My underlying response to The Four Burners Theory was to look for an approach to sidestep it. "Would i be able to succeed and keep each of the four burners running?" I pondered.

Maybe I could consolidate two burners. "Consider the possibility that I lumped loved ones into one classification.

Possibly I could consolidate wellbeing and work. "I hear sitting throughout the day is unfortunate. Consider the possibility that I got a standing work area?" Now, I realize what you are thinking. Accepting that you will be solid since you purchased a standing work area resembles trusting you are a revolutionary since you overlooked the attach safety belt sign on a plane, however whatever.

Before long I understood I was creating these workarounds on the grounds that I would not like to confront the main problem: life is loaded up with tradeoffs. In the event that you need to exceed expectations in your work and in your marriage, at that point your companions and your wellbeing may need to endure. On the off chance that you need to be solid and prevail as a parent, at that point you may be compelled to dial back your profession desire. Obviously, you are allowed to separate your time similarly among each of the four burners, yet you need to acknowledge that you will never arrive at your maximum capacity in some random zone.

Basically, we are compelled to pick. Okay rather carry on with a daily existence that is uneven, however high-acting in a specific territory? Or on the other hand would you rather carry on with a daily existence that is adjusted, however never boosts your potential in a given quadrant?

What is the most ideal approach to deal with these work-life balance issues? I don't profess to have it made sense of, yet here are three different ways of considering The Four Burners Theory.

Choice 1: Outsource Burners

We re-appropriate little parts of our carries on with constantly. We purchase inexpensive food so we don't need to cook. We go to the laundry to spare time on clothing. We visit the vehicle mechanics shop so we don't need to fix our own car.

Re-appropriating little segments of your life permits you to spare time and spend it somewhere else. Would you be able to apply similar plan to one quadrant of your life and save time to concentrate on the other three burners?

Work is the best model. For some, individuals, work is the most sizzling burner on the oven. It is the place they invest the most energy and it is the last burner to get killed. In principle, business people and entrepreneurs can redistribute the work burner. They do it by recruiting representatives.

In my article on The 3 Stages of Failure, I secured Sam Carpenter's tale about structure business frameworks that permitted him to work only 2 hours out of every week. He re-appropriated himself from the day by day work of the business while as yet receiving the money related rewards.

Child rearing is another model. Working guardians are regularly compelled to "re-appropriate" the family burner by dropping their youngsters off at childcare or recruiting a sitter. Calling this re-appropriating may appear to be uncalled for, yet—like the work model above—guardians are paying another person to keep the burner running while they utilize their time somewhere else.

The benefit of re-appropriating is that you can keep the burner running without investing your energy in it. Lamentably, eliminating yourself from the condition is likewise a drawback. Most business people, specialists, and makers I know would feel exhausted and without a feeling of direction on the off chance that they don't had anything to take a shot at every day. Each parent I know would prefer to invest energy with their youngsters than drop them off at childcare.

Re-appropriating keeps the burner running, yet is it running in a significant way?

Choice 2: Embrace Constraints

One of the most baffling pieces of The Four Burners Theory is that it sparkles a light on your undiscovered potential. It tends to be anything but difficult to think, "If just I had additional time, I could get more cash-flow or get fit as a fiddle or invest more energy at home."

One approach to deal with this issue is to move your concentration from wishing you had more opportunity to expanding the time you have. At the end of the day, you grasp your impediments. The inquiry to pose to yourself is, "Accepting a specific arrangement of requirements, how might I be as powerful as could reasonably be expected?"

For instance:

Expecting I can just work from 9 AM to 5 PM, how might I get the most cash-flow conceivable?

Expecting I can just compose for 15 minutes every day, how might I finish my book as quick as could be expected under the circumstances?

Accepting I can just exercise for 3 hours every week, how might I get in the most ideal shape?

This line of addressing pulls your concentration toward something positive (benefiting from what you have accessible) as opposed to something negative (stressing over failing to have sufficient opportunity). Besides, all around structured constraints can really improve your presentation and assist you with halting tarrying on your objectives.

Obviously, there are weaknesses too. Grasping requirements implies tolerating that you are working at not exactly your maximum capacity. Indeed, there are a lot of approaches to "work more efficiently" however it is hard to stay away from the way that where you invest your energy matters. On the off chance that you put additional time into your wellbeing or your connections or your profession, you would almost certainly observe improved outcomes here.

Alternative 3: The Seasons of Life

A third method to deal with your four burners is by breaking your life into seasons. Imagine a scenario in which, rather than looking for immaculate work-life balance consistently, you isolated your life into seasons that concentrated on a specific territory.

The significance of your burners may change all through life. At the point when you are in your 20s or 30s and you don't have youngsters, it tends to be simpler to get to the exercise center and pursue profession desire. The wellbeing and work burners are on to the max. A couple of years after the fact, you may begin a family and unexpectedly the wellbeing burner plunges down to a moderate stew while your family burner gets more gas. One more decade passes and you may restore associations with old companions or seek after that business thought you had been putting off.

You don't need to abandon your fantasies perpetually, however life seldom permits you to prop each of the four burners up without a moment's delay. Perhaps you have to relinquish something for this season. You can do it all in a lifetime, yet not at a similar damn time. In the expressions of Nathan Barry, "Focus on your objective with all that you have—for a season."

Besides, there is regularly a multiplier impact that happens when you devote yourself completely to a given zone. Much of the time, you can accomplish more by betting everything on a given undertaking for a couple of years than by giving it a tepid exertion for a long time. Possibly it is ideal to take a stab at periods of awkwardness and pivot through them varying.

Warren Buffett's "2 List" Strategy: How to Maximize Your Focus and Master Your Priorities

With well more than 50 billion dollars to his name, Warren Buffett is reliably positioned among the wealthiest individuals on the planet. Out of the apparent multitude of speculators in the twentieth century, Buffett was the best.

Given his prosperity, it makes sense that Buffett has a fantastic comprehension of how to invest his energy every day. From a money related point of view, you could state that he deals with his time better than any other individual.

What's more, that is the reason the story underneath, which was shared straightforwardly from Buffett's representative to my old buddy Scott Dinsmore, grabbed my eye.

We should discuss the basic 3-advance profitability system that Warren Buffett uses to enable his workers to decide their needs and activities.

The Story of Mike Flint

Mike Flint was Buffett's own plane pilot for a long time. (Rock has likewise flown four US Presidents, so I figure we can securely say he is acceptable at his specific employment.) According to Flint, he was discussing his vocation needs with Buffett when his supervisor requested that the pilot experience a 3-advance exercise.

Here's the means by which it works…

Stage 1: Buffett began by requesting that Flint record his main 25 vocation objectives. Along these lines, Flint took some time and kept in touch with them down. (Note: you could likewise finish this activity with objectives for a shorter course of events. For instance, record the main 25 things you need to achieve this week.)

Stage 2: Then, Buffett requested that Flint audit his rundown and circle his best 5 objectives. Once more, Flint took some time, cleared his path through the rundown, and in the long run settled on his 5 most significant objectives.

Note: If you're tracking with at home, stop at the present time and do these initial two stages before proceeding onward to Step 3.

Stage 3: At this point, Flint had two records. The 5 things he had surrounded were List An and the 20 things he had not orbited were List B.

Rock affirmed that he would begin dealing with his best 5 objectives immediately. What's more, that is when Buffett gotten some information about the subsequent rundown, "And shouldn't something be said about the ones you didn't circle?"

Stone answered, "Well, the main 5 are my essential center, however the other

20 arrive in a nearby second. They are as yet significant so I'll take a shot at those discontinuously as I see fit. They are not as dire, yet I despite everything intend to give them a devoted exertion."

To which Buffett answered, "No. You have it wrong, Mike. All that you didn't circle just turned into your Avoid-At-All-Cost list. Regardless, these things get no consideration from you until you've prevailing with your best 5."

The Power of Elimination

I have confidence in moderation and straightforwardness. I like disposing of waste. I imagine that dispensing with the inessential is perhaps the most ideal approaches to make life simpler, make great propensities more programmed, and make you appreciative for what you do have.

All things considered, disposing of inefficient things and choices is generally simple. It's taking out things you care about that is troublesome. It is difficult to forestall utilizing your time on things that are anything but difficult to support, yet that have little result. The assignments that have the best probability of wrecking your advancement are the ones you care about, however that aren't really significant.

Each conduct has an expense. Indeed, even unbiased practices aren't generally nonpartisan. They occupy time, vitality, and space that could be put toward better practices or more significant errands. We are frequently turning moving as opposed to making a move.

This is the reason Buffett's technique is especially splendid. Things 6 through 25 on your rundown are things you care about. They are critical to you. It is anything but difficult to legitimize investing your energy in them. Yet, when you contrast them with your main 5 objectives, these things are interruptions. Investing energy in auxiliary needs is the explanation you have 20 half-completed tasks rather than 5 finished ones.

Dispose of savagely. Power yourself to center. Complete an errand or murder it.

The most risky interruptions are the ones you love, however that don't cherish you back

The Difference Between Urgent and Important

What is significant is only here and there earnest and what is dire is only occasionally significant.

- Dwight Eisenhower

Critical assignments are things that you sense that you have to respond to: messages, calls, messages, reports. In the interim, in the expressions of Brett McKay, "Significant undertakings are things that add to our drawn out mission, qualities, and objectives."

Isolating these distinctions is sufficiently straightforward to do once, however doing so ceaselessly can be extreme. The explanation I like the Eisenhower Matrix is that it gives a reasonable structure to settling on the choices again and again. Furthermore, such as anything throughout everyday life, consistency is the crucial step.

Here are some different perceptions I've produced using utilizing this strategy.

Disposal Before Optimization

A couple of years back, I was finding out about PC programming when I went over a fascinating statement:

"There is no code quicker than no code."

– Kevlin Henney

At the end of the day, the quickest method to complete something — regardless of whether it is having a PC read a line of code or check an assignment off your plan for the day — is to kill that task totally. There is no quicker method to accomplish something than not doing it by any means. That is not motivation to be sluggish, yet rather a proposal to compel yourself to settle on hard choices and erase any undertaking that doesn't lead you toward your crucial, values, and your objectives.

Over and over again, we use profitability, time the board, and enhancement as a reason to evade the extremely troublesome inquiry: "Do I really should do this?" It is a lot simpler to stay occupied and reveal to yourself that you simply should be somewhat more effective or to "work a little later today" than to bear the agony of disposing of an assignment that you are OK with doing, however that isn't the most elevated and best utilization of your time.

As Tim Ferriss says, "Being occupied is a type of sluggishness — lethargic reasoning and unpredictable activity."

I find that the Eisenhower Matrix is especially helpful on the grounds that it pushes me to address whether an activity is extremely fundamental, which means I'm bound to move assignments to the "Erase" quadrant instead of carelessly rehashing them. What's more, to be completely forthright, on the off chance that you basically disposed of everything you sit around idly on every day then you presumably wouldn't require any tips on the best way to be more gainful at the things that issue.

Instructions to Build New Habits by Taking Advantage of Old Ones

In 2007, analysts at Oxford University began peering into the cerebrums of infants. What they discovered was astounding.

In the wake of contrasting the infant cerebrums with the typical grown-up human, the specialists understood that the normal grown-up had 41 percent less neurons than the normal infant.

From the outset, this disclosure didn't bode well. In the event that infants have more neurons, at that point for what reason are grown-ups more brilliant and more gifted?

We should discuss what is happening here, why this is significant, and what it has to improve propensities and acing your psychological and physical exhibition.

The Power of Synaptic Pruning

There is a wonder that occurs as we age called synaptic pruning. Neurotransmitters are associations between the neurons in your mind. The fundamental thought is that your mind prunes away associations between neurons that don't get utilized and develops associations that get utilized all the more oftentimes.

For instance, on the off chance that you work on playing the piano for a long time, at that point your mind will fortify the associations between those melodic neurons. The more you play, the more grounded the associations become. Not just that, the associations become quicker and more proficient each time you practice. As your mind constructs more grounded and quicker associations between neurons, you can communicate your abilities without breaking a sweat and skill. It is a natural change that prompts expertise advancement.

In the interim, another person who has never played the piano isn't reinforcing those associations in their mind. Subsequently, the cerebrum prunes away those unused associations and designates vitality toward building associations for other fundamental abilities.

This clarifies the contrast between infant minds and grown-up cerebrums. Children are brought into the world with cerebrums that resemble a clear canvas. Everything is a chance, however they don't have solid associations anyplace. The grown-ups, in any case, have pruned away a decent arrangement of their neurons, yet they have solid associations that help certain abilities.

Presently for the great part. We should discuss how synaptic pruning assumes a significant job in building new propensities.

Propensity Stacking

Synaptic pruning happens with each propensity you manufacture. As we've secured, your cerebrum constructs a solid system of neurons to help your present practices. The more you accomplish something, the more grounded and more proficient the association becomes.

You presumably have exceptionally solid propensities and associations that you underestimate every day. For instance, your mind is presumably exceptionally productive at making sure to scrub down every morning or to mix your morning mug of espresso or to open the blinds when the sun rises … or a large number of other day by day propensities. You can exploit these solid associations with assemble new propensities.

How?

With regards to building new propensities, you can utilize the connectedness of conduct for your potential benefit. Probably the most ideal approaches to manufacture another propensity is to recognize a current propensity you as of now do every day and afterward stack your new conduct on top. This is called propensity stacking.

Propensity stacking is a unique type of a usage aim. As opposed to blending your new propensity with a specific time and area, you pair it with a current propensity. This strategy, which was made by BJ Fogg as a major aspect of his Tiny Habits program, can be utilized to structure an undeniable sign for almost any propensity.

Propensity Stacking Examples

The propensity stacking recipe is:

After/Before [CURRENT HABIT], I will [NEW HABIT].

For instance:

After I pour some espresso every morning, I will contemplate for one moment.

After I remove my work shoes, I will quickly change into my exercise garments.

After I plunk down to supper, I will say one thing I'm thankful for that happened today.

After I get into bed around evening time, I will give my accomplice a kiss.

After I put on my running shoes, I will message a companion or relative where I am running and how long it will take.

Once more, the explanation propensity stacking works so well is that your present propensities are as of now incorporated with your mind. You have examples and practices that have been reinforced over years. By connecting your new propensities to a cycle that is as of now incorporated with your mind, you make it almost certain that you'll adhere to the new conduct.

When you have aced this essential structure, you can start to make bigger stacks by fastening little propensities together. This permits you to exploit the regular energy that originates from one conduct driving into the following.

Your morning schedule propensity stack may resemble this:

After I pour my morning mug of espresso, I will think for sixty seconds.

After I think for sixty seconds, I will compose my daily agenda for the afternoon.

After I compose my plan for the day for the afternoon, I will promptly start my first assignment.

Or on the other hand, consider this propensity stack at night:

After I get done with having supper, I will put my plate straightforwardly into the dishwasher.

After I set my dishes aside, I will quickly wipe down the counter.

After I wipe down the counter, I will set out my espresso cup for tomorrow first thing.

You can likewise embed new practices into the center of your present schedules. For instance, you may as of now have a morning schedule that appears as though this: Wake up > Make my bed > Take a shower. Suppose you need to build up the propensity for perusing all the more every night. You can extend your propensity stack and take a stab at something like:

Wake up > Make my bed > Place a book on my pad > Take a shower. Presently, when you move into bed every night, a book will be staying there hanging tight for you to appreciate.

Generally speaking, propensity stacking permits you to make a lot of basic standards that manage your future conduct. It resembles you generally have a course of action for which activity should come straightaway. When you get settled with this methodology, you can create general propensity stacks to manage you at whatever point the circumstance is suitable:

At the point when I see a lot of steps, I will take them as opposed to utilizing the lift.

Social aptitudes. At the point when I stroll into a gathering, I will acquaint myself with anybody I don't have the foggiest idea yet.

At the point when I need to purchase something over $100, I will hold up 24 hours before buying.

Smart dieting. At the point when I serve myself a feast, I will consistently put veggies on my plate first.

At the point when I purchase another thing, I will part with something. ("One in, one out.")

At the point when the telephone rings, I will take one full breath and grin before replying.

At the point when I leave an open spot, I will check the table and seats to ensure I don't abandon anything.

Regardless of how you utilize this technique, the key to making a fruitful propensity stack is choosing the correct sign to kick things off. In contrast to a usage goal, which explicitly expresses the time and area for a given conduct, propensity stacking certainly has the opportunity and area incorporated with it. When and where you decide to embed a propensity into your day by day schedule can have a major effect. In case you're attempting to include reflection into your morning schedule yet mornings are clamorous and your children continue running into the room, at that point that might be an inappropriate spot and time. Consider when you are destined to be effective. Try not to request that yourself do a propensity when you're probably going to be busy with something different.

Your prompt ought to likewise have a similar recurrence as your ideal propensity. In the event that you need to do a propensity consistently, however you stack it on head of a propensity that just occurs on Mondays, that is not a decent decision.

Finding the Right Trigger

One approach to locate the correct trigger for your propensity stack is by conceptualizing a rundown of your present propensities. You can utilize your Habits Scorecard as a beginning stage. Then again, you can make a rundown with two sections. In the principal section, record the propensities you do every day no matter what.

For instance:

Get up.

Wash up.

Brush your teeth.

Get dressed.

Blend some espresso.

Have breakfast.

Take the children to class.

Start the work day.

Have lunch.

End the work day.

Change jobless garments.

Plunk down for supper.

Mood killer the lights.

Get into bed.

Your rundown can be any longer, yet you get the thought. In the subsequent section, record everything that transpire every day come what may. For instance:

The sun rises.

You get an instant message.

The melody you are tuning in to closes.

The sun sets.

Equipped with these two records, you can start looking for the best spot to layer your new propensity into your way of life.

Do Things You Can Sustain

In 1996, Southwest Airlines was confronted with an intriguing issue.

During the earlier decade, the aircraft organization had systematically extended from being a little provincial transporter to one with a more public nearness. Furthermore, presently, in excess of 100 urban communities were calling for Southwest to extend administration to their area. When numerous carrier organizations were losing cash or failing, Southwest was flooding with circumstance.

So what did they do?

Southwest turned down over 95% of the offers and started serving only 4 new areas in 1996. They left noteworthy development on the table.

For what reason would a business turn down so much chance? What's more, more significant, what would we be able to gain from this story and put to use in our own lives?

What Is Your Upper Bound?

Beginning during the 1970s, Southwest was the main carrier organization that made a benefit for almost 30 sequential years. In his book Great by Choice, writer Jim Collins guarantees that one of the key to Southwest's prosperity was the ability of organization pioneers to set an upper headed breaking point for development.

Indeed, Southwest chiefs needed to develop the business every year. However, they purposefully abstained from becoming excessively. The organization chiefs picked a pace that they could continue, so the business could develop while keeping up the way of life and gainfulness. They set an upper headed cutoff for their development.

This is a methodology that can be applied to almost any objective, business or something else. The vast majority, notwithstanding, will in general do the inverse and spotlight just on the lower bound.

An individual may state, "I need to lose in any event 5 pounds this month."

A business person may state, "I need to make in any event 10 deals calls today."

A craftsman may state, "I need to compose at any rate 500 words today."

A ball player may state, "I need to make at any rate 50 free tosses today."

We will in general spotlight just on the lower bound: the base limit we need to hit. What's more, the verifiable supposition that is, "Hello, in the event that you can accomplish more than the base, take the plunge."

However, what might it resemble in the event that we added an upper bound to our objectives and practices?

"I need to lose in any event 5 pounds this month, yet not more than 10."

"I need to make in any event 10 deals calls today, yet not more than 20."

"I need to compose at any rate 500 words today, however not more than 1,500."

"I need to make at any rate 50 free tosses today, however not more than 100."

In numerous everyday issues, there is an otherworldly zone of long haul development: Pushing enough to gain ground, however less that it is unreasonable.

Take, for instance, weightlifting .

Over the previous year, I have gradually added 5 pounds to my squat like clockwork. A year back, I began with a weight that was excessively light: 200 lbs. for 5 arrangements of 5 reps. A week ago, I completed 300 lbs. for 5 arrangements of 5 reps. I never followed a mysterious program. I basically accomplished the work and included 5 pounds like clockwork or something like that.

Certainly, as far as possible was significant. I needed to maintain adding weight in control to get more grounded. However, as far as possible was similarly as basic. I needed to develop gradually and deliberately on the off chance that I needed to forestall aggravation and injury. There were a lot of days when I could have included 10 pounds. Possibly 15 pounds. Yet, in the event that I forcefully sought after development I would have immediately hit a level (or more regrettable, caused a physical issue).

Rather, I picked remain inside a wellbeing edge of development and abstained from going excessively quick. I needed each set to feel simple.

The intensity of setting a furthest breaking point is that it gets simpler for you to continue your advancement. Furthermore, the intensity of continuing your advancement is that you wind up overwhelming each and every individual who pursued accomplishment as fast as could be expected under the circumstances.

Put another way: Average speed wins.

Do Things You Can Sustain

There is a straightforward method to incorporate this thought: Let upper bound cutoff points drive your practices to start with and afterward gradually increment your yield.

Let's assume you need to begin working out. A great many people would concentrate on as far as possible and state, "I need to begin practicing for at any rate 45 minutes on Monday, Wednesday, and Friday."

Rather, you could flip around the issue and state, "I am not permitted to practice for over 5 minutes on Monday, Wednesday, and Friday.

By setting a fantastically simple furthest cutoff, you make the way toward beginning and supporting your conduct a lot less difficult. When you build up the daily schedule of doing your conduct again and again, you can raise the cutoff varying.

It is smarter to gain little ground each day than to do as much as humanly conceivable in one day. Do things you can continue.

www.ingramcontent.com/pod-product-compliance
Lightning Source LLC
Chambersburg PA
CBHW030421160726
47992CB00007B/3227